ICU Nurse Notebook

nurse

{ners} n. a scrub wearing, smile bringing, life saving rockstar who lives to heal and loves to encourage.

See also: SUPERHERO

I0462478

This book belongs to:

_____

DATE: _____

DATE: _____

DATE: _____

DATE: _____

DATE: _____

DATE: _____

DATE: _____

DATE: _____

DATE: _____

DATE: _____

DATE: _____

DATE: _____

DATE: _____

DATE: _____

DATE: _____

DATE: _____

DATE: _____

DATE: _____

DATE: _____

DATE: _____

DATE: _____

DATE: _____

DATE: _____

DATE: _____

DATE: _____

DATE: _____

DATE: _____

DATE: _____

DATE: _____

DATE: _____

DATE: _____

DATE: _____

DATE: _____

DATE: _____

DATE: _____

DATE: _____

DATE: _____

DATE: _____

DATE: _____

DATE: _____

DATE: _____

DATE: _____

DATE: _____

DATE: _____

DATE: _____

DATE: _____

Quotes from Patients

Date

Who?

Where?

Quote

_____

_____

_____

_____

Quotes from Patients

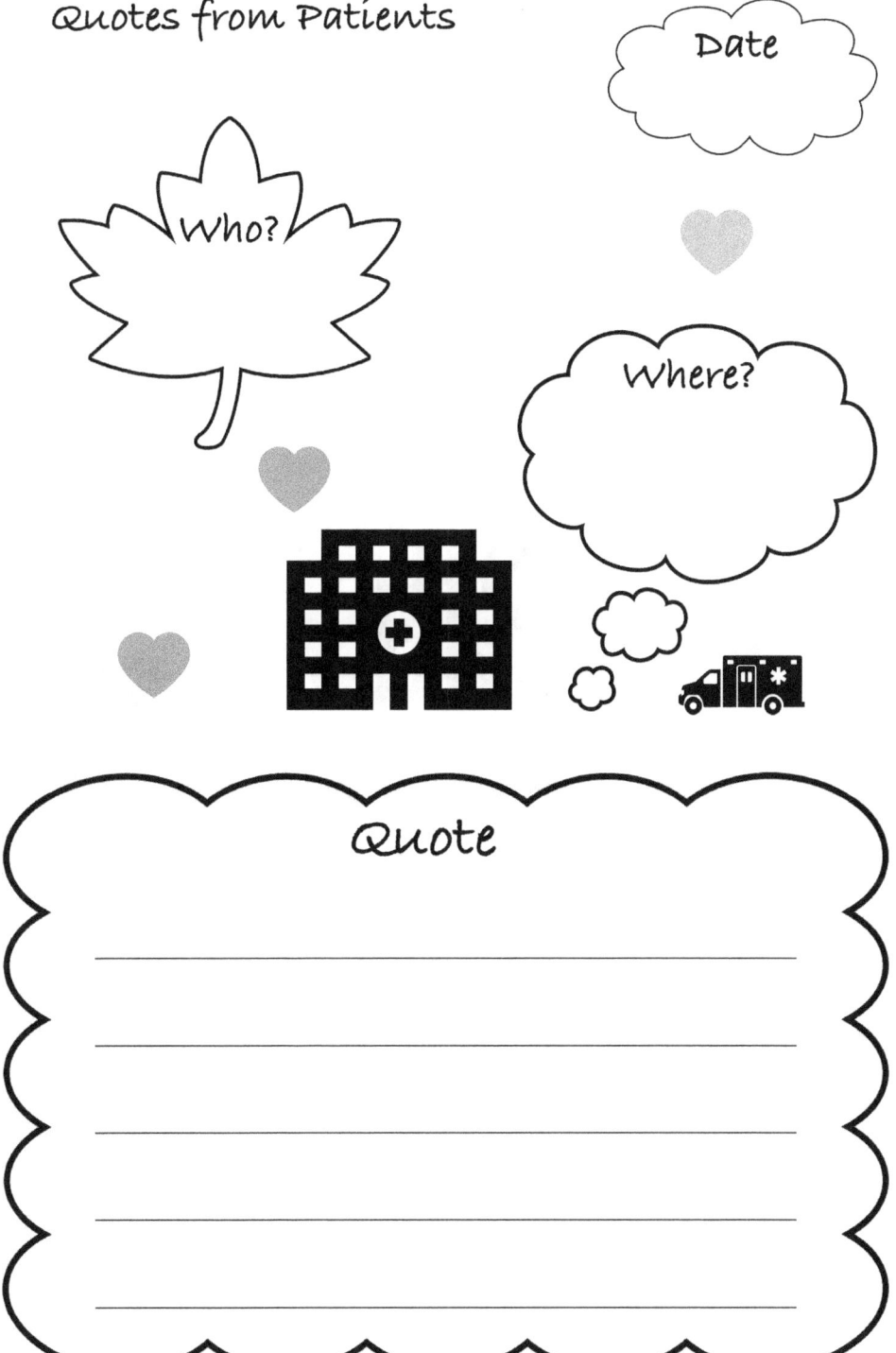

Date

Who?

Where?

Quote

_____
_____
_____
_____
_____

Quotes from Patients

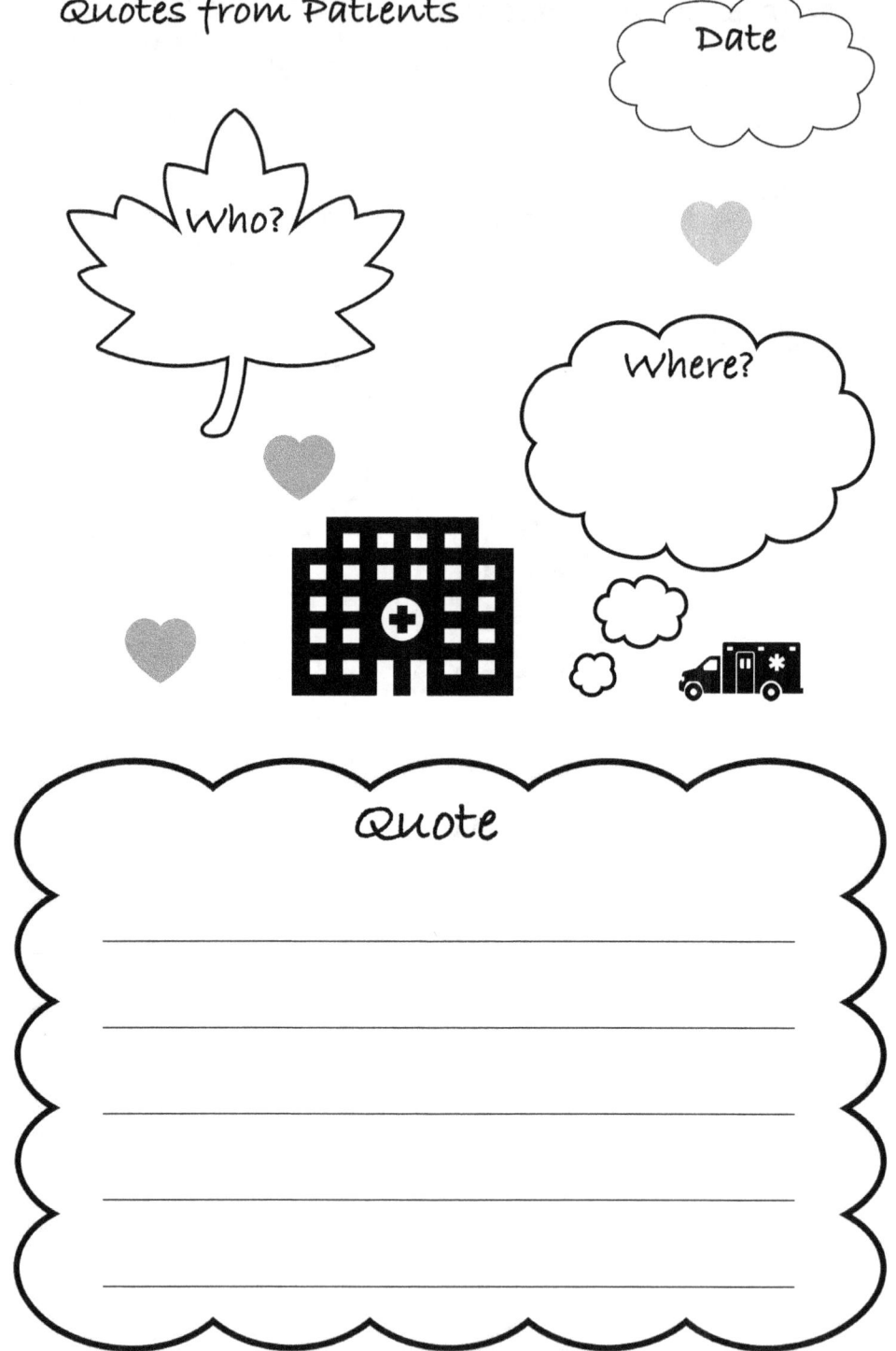

Date

Who?

Where?

Quote

Quotes from Patients

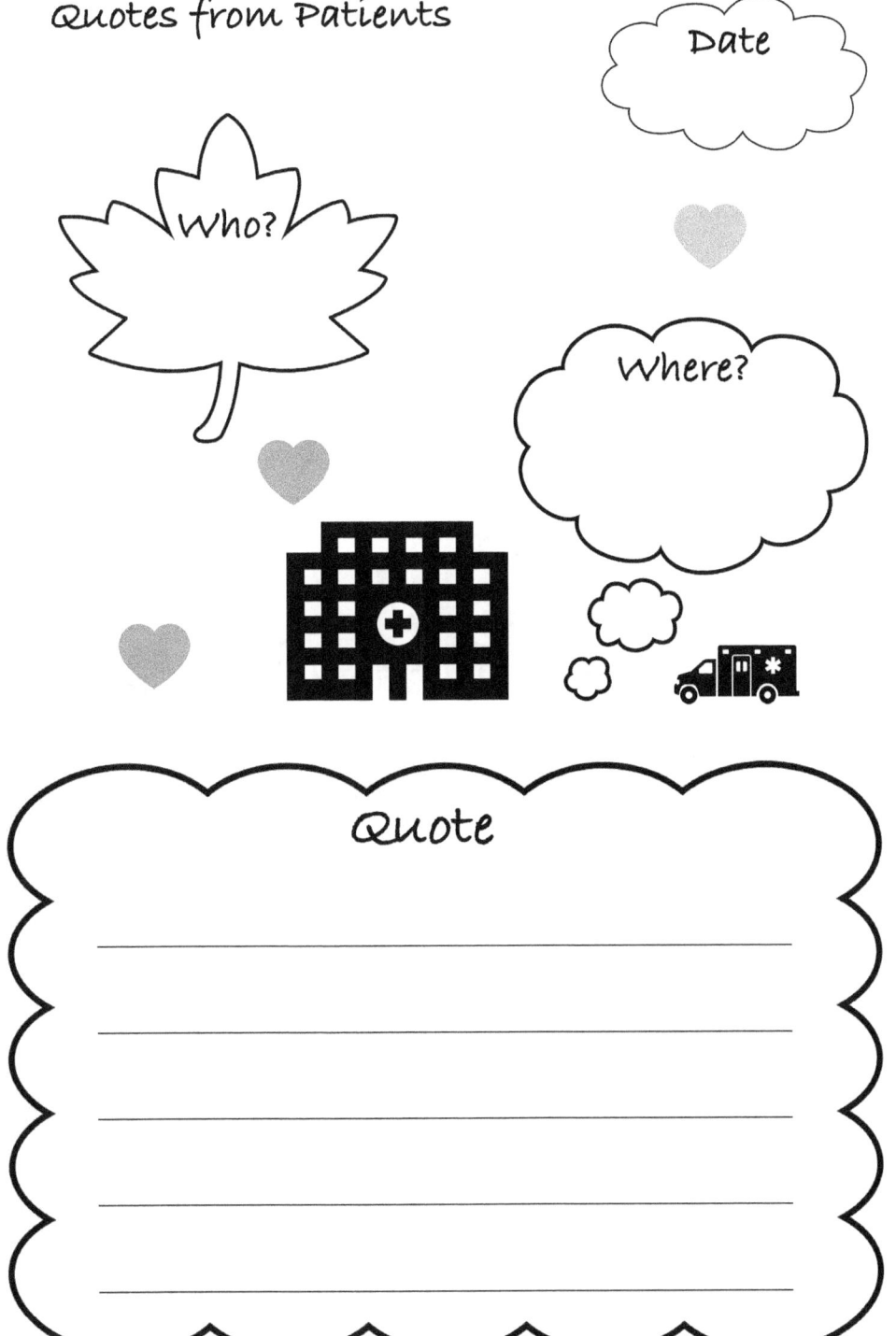

Date

Who?

Where?

Quote

Quotes from Patients

Date

Who?

Where?

Quote

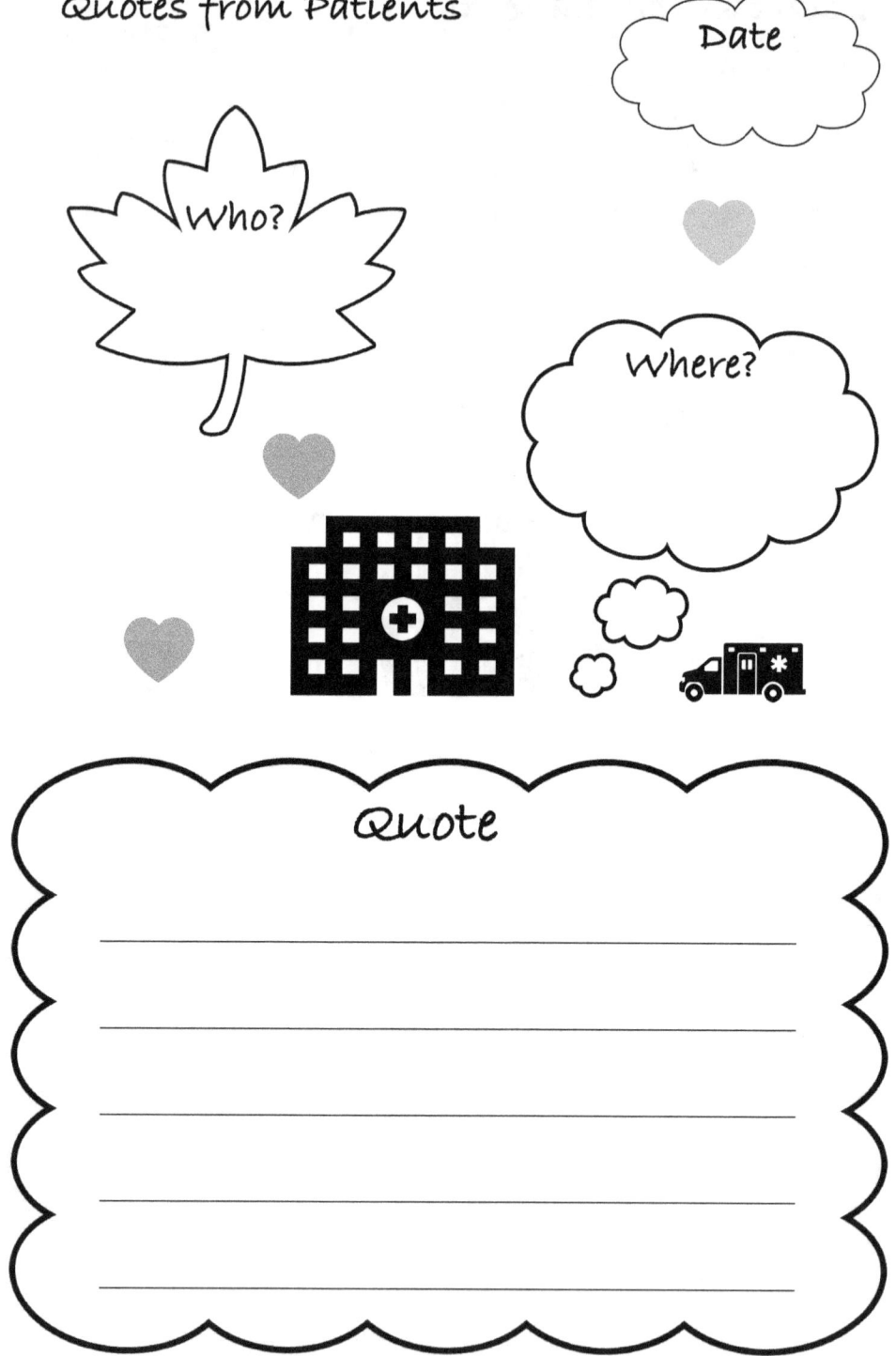

Coloring Section

I Had Fun Once, Then
I Went To Nursing School

Ativan A Nurse's Best Friend

Eat.
Sleep.
Nurse.
Repeat

DO NOT MAKE ME SEDATE YOU.

Best Nurse Ever

I'VE SEEN MORE
PRIVATES
THAN THE ARMY
GENERAL

Nurse Squad

If You're Happy and You Know It, It's Your Meds

www.ingramcontent.com/pod-product-compliance
Lightning Source LLC
Chambersburg PA
CBHW072153170526
45158CB00004BA/1634